ANXIETY

Self Management

FREE YOUR LIFE AND OVERCOME ANXIETY, FEAR AND PANIC ATTACKS

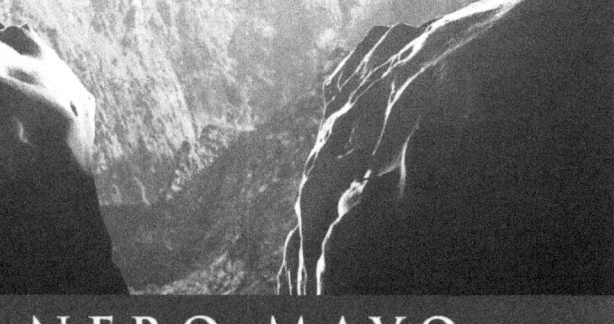

NERO MAYO

Anxiety Self-Management in English

Free THANK YOU Offer

Before I dive in to the good stuff I want to be a little transparent. I don't just want to provide you one book that you get a hold of, and that is that. I want to have people, like you, that I notify when I'm putting out other valuable content. Your thinking, "what's in it for me?" Well, if you get a hold of it early it'll probably be free. This right-

At the end of this book you will find a link to the author page. This will give you the opportunity to join my email list and as a result, notifications of future releases as well as free content and discounts!

Introduction

All of us have stress. This is normal. Stress combined with fear creates anxiety. Anxiety is a devilish little monster. It can take control of your life. Anxiety can cost you your career, your relationships, and even the simplicity of living a fulfilling life. Anxiety robs you of the drive to take chances and you miss out on seeing where those chances will take you.

Although not much has been proven about anxiety, managing it is actually possible. With the right information and enough determination, you'll be able to get rid of stress and start living the life you have the right to live. Anxiety does not have to be part of your daily life. After reading and implementing the steps in this Ebook Anxiety will no longer prevent you from the activities you enjoy, the people you care about or the jobs that fulfil your unique talents.

Chapter 1: Understanding the Basic

Anxiety. What is it?

Anxiety is often a confusing and frustrating feeling. Fear is the normal physiological reaction against threat apprehension while worry is normal reaction against distress. Not a lot of people understand what anxiety is. Some people take it as a sign that something is wrong with them, while there are others who are more preoccupied with the symptoms such as heart palpitations and shortness of breath. There are also people who see it as a sign of weakness or mental disease.

The sad truth is it's these misconceptions that make it even harder for people to understand anxiety. Instead of finding ways to deal with it, people feel discouraged to ask for any form of help. Understanding Anxiety is crucial to managing it.

The first step to managing anxiety is awareness. In order to understand anxiety, you first need to know how to recognize it properly. There's no way that you'll be able to solve a problem without knowing the facts first.

Reading about anxiety can already be intimidating so it's important that have the right information. By knowing exactly what you're dealing with, you'll be able to have a better grasp of what anxiety really is. You won't feel confused or ashamed that you have episodic anxiety attacks. You'll realize that there really is nothing wrong with you and that with the right information; you'll be able to manage those anxiety attacks successfully.

But before you can get started on dealing with those anxiety attacks, you need to understand 2 important truths.

One, anxiety is normal, and

two, anxiety is a response.

Everyone goes through times of anxiety. No matter how deep in an anxiety attack you think you are, find comfort in knowing that it's manageable and the more you can manage without medication or substances- the stronger you will become in dealing with future episodes. Anxiety is just a part of life.

Anxiety is our body's response to something that poses a particular threat or danger. Think of it as an alarm system that pushes the body to go into fight or flight mode. When anxiety starts to creep in, your body's adrenaline rush is triggered. This then signals the body to start preparing for defense.

Even though anxiety feels uncomfortable overall, it's really just your body's fight or flight mechanism taking over. There's really no reason for you to feel afraid or confused when you suddenly feel the 'alarm reaction'.

EVERYONE has anxiety

In trying to overcome anxiety, there will be times when you will get bogged down by negative thoughts. There will be days when you beat yourself up over particular stressors but it is important that you keep yourself level headed Mediation daily can help considerably.

Let's face it. It's hard to think positively 24/7. When we let anxiety take over, the world suddenly turns into a threatening place to live. You don't see it for what it is. You just let how it makes you feel control you, and this is where the real danger starts. It's when you allow your thoughts to hijack your reality that it becomes hard to cope with anxiety.

So how do you nip anxiety in the bud? By replacing all the negative thoughts with realistic thoughts. Separating yourself from the situation and taking a step back and looking at the entire picture before you make any conclusions. Think of it as "viewing the situation through third person." If you were playing a video game or suggesting to someone else how to get through an episode. It's when you take an unbiased look into the situation that you will realize that the emotions that seem "out-of-control" are actually manageable.

The Different Types of Anxiety

According to the *Diagnostic and Statistical Manual of Mental Disorders, Fifth Edition (DSM-5)*, a book published by the American Psychiatric Association, and accepted as valid worldwide by mental health professionals, the primary types of anxiety disorders are specific phobia, social anxiety disorder, panic disorder, generalized anxiety disorder, and agoraphobia.

Agoraphobia

The person with agoraphobia is afraid of being out in the open, such as being in the middle of a parking lot or a supermarket. (Or being in the middle of a supermarket parking lot.) They are often afraid of using public transportation because people with agoraphobia fear such closeness. Crowds are terrifying to the agoraphobic person.

Agoraphobia may prevent someone from keeping a job other than a home-based one, and consequently, they must prevail upon others to bring them food, water, and the other necessities of life. Even walking to the mailbox at the end of the driveway to retrieve the mail may be well beyond the capability of the agoraphobic person. Fortunately, agoraphobia, as with the other anxiety disorders, is treatable.

Specific phobia

The person with a specific phobia fears a particular type of object, such as spiders or snakes. Of course, many people fear snakes and spiders, but the phobic person suffers an extreme fear that extends well beyond that of the average person.

Some phobias seem very silly to people, such as the fear of frogs (batrachophobia), of chickens (alektorophobia) or of bats (chiroptophobia). Most people don't encounter frogs or live chickens in their daily lives, and certainly you can easily avoid bats (unless you enter their caves or other locations where bats like to hang out). The phobia may become so intense that the person avoids large areas where they believe that the feared object might be, like a street, city, or even a province or state where the person once saw a frog, in the case of the batrachophobic person.

Panic disorder

Panic disorder is characterized by frequent and chronic panic attacks. A panic attack is a type of debilitating anxiety that overwhelms and overcomes the person on a regular basis. She feels as if she is dying, although she might not know why she has this fear.

A panic attack is often accompanied by an increased heart rate and blood pressure, and many people in the midst of a panic attack think they are having a heart attack or stroke with a panic attack. Super cold sweats, crying and uncontrollable short rapid breaths occur in severe attacks. Fortunately, panic attacks can be treated with deep breathing as well as with medication, herbal remedies, and many other options, all described in this book.

Generalized anxiety disorder (GAD)

If you have generalized anxiety disorder (GAD), you probably know that you frequently have an overwhelming sense of dread and impending doom, but you don't know what it is that you fear so much. This is a very scary and also a very frustrating experience.

For the person with GAD, almost everything is experienced as an "Oh, no!" event. Even if something wonderful happens, like you get a pay raise or fall in love with your soulmate, the person with GAD worries that this was such a great thing that happened, that it must be balanced out by some terrible event. This is not rational thinking and it puts a damper over the person's whole life. Fortunately, GAD is highly treatable, as are all forms of anxiety disorders.

Social anxiety disorder (SAD)

Nearly everyone can remember a time when they had to give a presentation or speak up in church or elsewhere. The fear of public speaking is a nearly universal one. Organizations like Toastmasters help people to reverse their anxiety over speaking in public.

Social anxiety disorder (SAD) goes far beyond common everyday social fears. With this disorder, the person becomes anxious and fearful about interacting with nearly everyone, anywhere, with the exception of parents and very close friends.

He worries that he is highly likely to say something stupid or embarrassing, while she thinks that she might trip and fall down, and everyone will laugh at her. In fact, he and she can see such terrible events happening in their minds. The person is so afraid of doing something catastrophic that he or she foregoes nearly all social contact. As a result of this disorder, these individuals are often very lonely people.

Chapter 2 Pharmaceuticals that are common in 2016

There are many therapies available for people who suffers different types of anxiety. These therapies accompanied by anti- anxiety drugs will greatly improve the life of people who suffer from this disorder. Therapy often helps people who have anxiety disorders, although the type of therapy that is used may vary.

Typically when someone doesn't know they have a form of anxiety usually it is triggered and they find themselves in a compromising situation. Shortly after this episode they are diagnosed and spend time in inpatient care before transitioning into a long term outpatient therapy program. The most common form of therapy that is used today is called cognitive-behavioral therapy (CBT). This form of therapy helps people identify and challenge the irrational beliefs that are key to their disorder. However, some anxiety disorders are treated with exposure therapy, in which they are gradually helped to think about, and eventually face, the objects that they fear.

A combination of therapies may also be helpful, such as CBT and exposure therapy or other forms of therapy. Group therapy can help individuals with anxiety disorders considerably, because they learn that they are not the only ones suffering with anxiety, and thus they may feel less alone as others share their symptoms, their fears, and also their successes.

Exposure Therapy

Exposure therapy is commonly used with phobic individuals. Exposure therapy refers to a slow but steadily increasing exposure to the feared object. At first, the person learns to *think* about the feared thing, and in the course of thinking about it, she is trained to relax and calm her feelings of anxiety.

Later, if it is possible and practical, the person is exposed at a distance to the feared object, such as a dog or a horse. Of course if a person is deathly afraid of tigers, the closest they will get to this type of animal is within a safe distance from a cage in the zoo. Tigers really are dangerous.

Interestingly, research has shown that when a person can relax while thinking about something that's normally scary for him (the phobic object), those relaxed feelings actually remain with him later on when he's at a safe distance from the feared object. It's as if both the body and mind have become desensitized to their former fear factor.

Keep in mind, however, that in times of extreme stress, the former phobia may recur, and exposure therapy will be needed again.

Cognitive-Behavioral Therapy (CBT)

Cognitive-behavioral therapy (CBT) is an evidence-based therapy, which means that research has shown that this type of therapy is highly effective in helping many people.

With CBT, the therapist talks to clients and learns what is going on in their lives. Once sufficient information has been gained, the therapist helps clients identify the key underlying irrational beliefs, sometimes referred to as thought distortions. These thought distortions are causing major problems in their lives. Then the person learns to recognize thoughts expressing irrational beliefs and challenge these beliefs in her own mind.

One common thought distortion is an all or nothing thinking, also sometimes called black and white thinking. The person with this type of an irrational belief thinks that everything is either terrible or it is wonderful. There are no gray areas and no middle ground. Yet much of life really is sort of neutral—not fabulous and not terrible.

Catastrophizing is another type of irrational thinking that the CBT therapist helps a person challenge. The person misses breakfast, and may think, that's it, my whole day is ruined now. And her whole day probably *is* ruined, but only because of her irrational thinking, which will cause her to see everything through a dark and unhappy prism. The person with an anxiety disorder may take catastrophic thoughts to an extreme level, seeing death, severe injury or financial ruin around every corner.

The fallacy of fairness is a very common thought distortion, or the belief that life "should" be fair. People may think, I'm a good person, so why do I have this stupid anxiety disorder? The reality is that having a psychological problem is not related to being good or bad. Nice people have anxiety disorders and so do some not-so-nice people. Bad things happen to good people.

CBT therapists often may employ deep breathing and progressive muscle relaxation therapies to help their anxious clients. The reason for using these techniques is that the anxious person often experiences rapid and panicked breathing and an excessive tightening of the muscles. Read more about these two techniques in Chapter 6.

Group Therapy

Many people benefit from individual therapy, but group therapy can also be extremely helpful. When people who suffer from a common or related problem meet as a group, they learn that they do not suffer alone, as so many had assumed that they did. They also learn to share experiences and give and take suggestions from others.

Chapter 3: Natural Remedies for Anxiety

Managing your Anxiety shouldn't cost you anything but the right mindset. You do not need to spend thousands of dollars to relieve your anxiety. Nature offers plenty of remedies that can help calm your mind. Studies have shown that some herbal remedies may help you to resolve your anxiety, at least temporarily. For example, Valerian is one herb that sometimes is used to treat anxiety, and Chamomile is another. Lavender is also an herbal remedy, but it is primarily used as a form of aromatherapy, a subject that is covered in Chapter 5.

Before you take any herb or supplement for any reason whatsoever, first check with your doctor to make sure that it would be safe for you and will not interact with other medications that you take. Do not assume that because a drug is natural, that this means that it is also safe. Cobra venom is also natural—but you wouldn't want it injected into you.

You can purchase most herbal remedies in supermarkets or pharmacies or you may wish to order them online. Never take more than the amount recommended by your doctor or on the package. If the package says to take one pill a day, do not assume you'll feel better four times faster if you take four pills a day. When it comes to drugs, including herbal remedies (which act on the body similarly to drugs), more isn't necessarily better.

COMBINATIONS OF HERBAL REMEDIES

Sometimes sellers of herbal remedies combine two or more herbs into one capsule or tablet. For example, as mentioned, a sleep remedy may contain both Valerian and Chamomile or other combinations of herbs. Always read the labels. If you are already taking sedating medications, such as an over-the-counter or prescribed medication, stay away from herbal remedy combinations until you can check with your doctor.

VALERIAN

Valerian, or *Valeriana officinalis,* is an herbal remedy that is sometimes used to help individuals suffering from anxiety and/or insomnia. However, there is not enough research to date to verify whether Valerian is effective in helping anxiety or not. This herbal remedy may cause stomach aches and headaches in some individuals.

Valerian is sometimes combined in tablets along with Chamomile. Combined medications, even when they are "natural," should be used with caution. Never consume alcohol or take any other sedating drugs with any of the herbs described in this chapter.

GINKGO

Some research indicates that supplements of the herb ginkgo (*ginkgo biloba*) may improve anxiety in suffering individuals, although larger studies are needed to confirm this finding. This herbal remedy may cause stomachache, nausea, and diarrhea in some individuals (even moreso if taken on an empty stomach. In addition, people taking blood thinners should avoid this herb altogether, because the blood may become too thin with ginkgo.

LEMON BALM

Also available as a form of aromatherapy, lemon balm (*Melissa officinalis*) has been shown helpful in reducing anxiety in some small studies Sometimes lemon balm is combined with chamomile. This herbal remedy may be available as a capsule or a tea.

PASSIONFLOWER

Passionflower, also known in Latin as *Passiflora incarnate*, is a plant that has sometimes been used to help people suffering with anxiety or depression. Passionflower is available in tablets, a liquid form, and as capsules. Research has shown some efficacy on anxiety with this remedy.

According to the National Center for Complementary and Integrative Health, a federal government agency in the United States, passionflower may cause drowsiness. Of course if you have a problem with insomnia, as many anxious people do, you might consider this side effect to be a benefit instead of a side effect.

CHAMOMILE

Chamomile has been used for many years to help people with stomach aches and diarrhea, as well as with anxiety. Some researchers at the University of Pennsylvania reported their findings on the effects of chamomile on people with anxiety in 2009. They found that chamomile significantly decreased the anxiety levels of their subjects, all of whom had been diagnosed with mild to moderate generalized anxiety disorder (GAD).

Chamomile is available as a tablet, capsule or a liquid extract or this herb can be taken in a tea. There are different types of chamomile, but most people favor German chamomile. Some people are allergic to chamomile, especially those individuals who are also allergic to ragweed or daisies, since these plants are related.

ST. JOHN'S WORT

The herb St. John's wort, also known as *Hypericum perforatum*, is sometimes used to decrease both depression and anxiety. It is one of the oldest medicinal herbs known. However, some people may develop anxiety as a result of using St. John's wort. So far, only one small study in Germany found that St. John's wort improved anxiety, although effective.

It should be noted that St. John's wort reacts with many different types of medications, such as antidepressants, some heart medicines, and birth control pills, to name just a few. This is why it's very important to avoid this herb until you've first checked with your physician, received approval in advance, and you are aware of any possible interactions with other medications you take.

RHODIOLA

Rhodiola (*Rhodiola rosea)* is sometimes used to treat anxiety, as well as headache, fatigue, and depression. The root extracts of this plant are available in capsules or tablets, as well as in a tea form. There is no research to date on the effects of Rhodiola on anxiety just documented accounts.

SKULLCAP

Some limited research indicates that the Chinese skullcap plant (*Scutellaria baicalensis*) may have some anti-anxiety qualities, although further research is needed. There is also an American form of skullcap, also known as *Scutellaria lateriflora*.

The American skullcap is available as a liquid extract or a powder, while the Chinese skullcap is only available in a powdered form.

People with diabetes should avoid taking this herbal remedy because it may increase the risk for low blood sugar (hypoglycemia). This herb should not be taken with barbiturates or benzodiazepine medications or with any drugs used to treat insomnia. It should also be avoided in people taking anti-seizure medications.

GREEN TEA

Some small studies have found that green tea reduces anxiety levels, but much more research is needed before green tea can be validated as a good antidote for anxiety. Keep in mind that green tea includes caffeine, so this substance could increase the risk for anxiety. There are some indications that the liver may be negatively affected by green tea. Further studies should provide additional information.

Chapter 4: Breathing and meditation techniques

Almost everyone wishes to have a life that's free of stress, but no one can escape stress. Some may even say that it is already a lifestyle. The young generation nowadays is more health conscious and values a sound body, mind, and spirit. That's the reason why there have been many research studies that evolved to attempt to know the techniques that will work to combat stress.

It's best to be open minded, enough to see the advantages that one will benefit. It will be an opportunity to reflect on oneself in respond to stress, and to check on one's stress tolerance. After all, the main reason why certain techniques have evolved is all because of stress.

Stress is a normal physical reaction when one can sense an event as a threat which causes or upsets the balance of one's mind and body. It is somewhat like an automatic "push button" as a defense when our body senses danger, whether it is perceived as real or imagined.

Breathing Techniques to Start

Controlled deep breathing is one technique being taught by Buddhists in their meditation classes. Meditation is a great gift that you can give to your mind and to your well-being. It is a time for you and you alone. It is the best exercise that you can give to yourself. The ultimate goal is to create calmness and acceptance as you let thoughts come and go without getting stuck in them.

There are a few different Breathing techniques being taught in basic Meditation classes. This is a way to calm your mind and become aware of the breathing. Here are some, to name a few:

1. Just sit. A quiet place is preferred.

2. Close your eyes and focus as you inhale and exhale.

3. Just relax as you breathe. Don't try to control your breathing. Just breathe naturally.

4. When your mind starts to wander off, just make sure that you'll bring your awareness back to your breathing.

5. There's no need to get frustrated when your mind starts to wander off. Be kind to yourself.

6. Prolonged sitting for a period of time isn't necessary.

7. Five minutes of your quiet time will do. Just relax and be patient.

8. Be in a comfortable position, like lying on your back or sitting.

9. Just make sure that if you're sitting that you should keep your spine straight and simply drop your shoulders in a relaxed manner.

10. Close your eyes.

11. Bring your attention to your abdomen as you feel it rise and expand as you inhale and exhale.

12. Your focus of attention is on the duration of your breathing, as if you are on your surfing board riding through the waves of your breath as you inhale and exhale.

13. When your mind starts to wander off, then always make sure to bring your focus and attention back to your breathing.

14. Do this for 20 minutes per day. I personally do it more than once a day.

Why Meditation Works

When you meditate, you are able to focus entirely on the present moment because you cease from thinking about your   personal   worries, anxieties, work deadlines, and daily tasks.

During meditation, you are able to silence your mental clutter. This leads to a state of complete relaxation of your mind.

The transformations experienced by the mind and body during meditation can be quantified scientifically. During the state of relaxation brought about by meditation both the heart rate and respiration are significantly slowed down. It has also been discovered that the frequency of the brain waves is decelerated during meditation.

When you are functioning at your normal level of consciousness your brain waves run at 13 to 30 cycles each second. This is dramatically reduced to 8 to 13 cycles per second during the meditative state.

Chapter 5: Activities You Can Try

Socialization

Anxiety and depression worsen when left ignored. Socializing gives you opportunity to let them be addressed. Let other people in and make new happy memories to counter your worries. Give yourself time to explore the world because all the negatives are just one part of it.

Attend parties. Go window shopping or actual shopping if you have the budget. Get a date. See a movie. Make new friends to stand as your personal support group. Socialization can be nice if you focus on fun.

Exercise

In the past, almost all exercises are recommended as some sort of anxiety relief. The body's serotonergic system that has a direct link to anxiety and depression, becomes more active when you exercise. Its higher activity stimulates the brain to produce more endorphins and minimize the production of cortisol and adrenaline. Another benefit of exercising is the increased amount of oxygen in the brain, which makes it more efficient in thinking and processing.

However, according to The Center for Emotional Health of Greater Philadelphia, LLC, it is not enough to make exercising a habit because it needs to be a physical and emotional activity at the same time. Exercising needs to be comforting, relaxing and fun. It may not be of great help if you force yourself to exercise even if you feel bad about it because it defeats the purpose.

Maura Mulligan from the Center for Wellness at Wentworth Institute of Technology recommends doing light exercises for an hour five times a week. This is to warm you up for a more active lifestyle ahead. Eventually though, you have to stick with physical activities that you enjoy and have meaning to you.

For instance, instead of adopting a general exercise routine in the gym or from TV, think about the strengths and hobbies that you can apply. Make dancing your exercise if you are good at it or play your favorite sport if you are into it. You need to be happy and confident in what you do to really benefit from it.

You can also try to remember what you used to have fun with as a child. Activities that you used to do as a child have deeper emotional connection to you, provided that your childhood is what people call normal and healthy.

Another way to figure out the most suitable physical activity for you is to determine your interests and the things you have always wanted to try. Excitement helps because it is a good feeling. Naturally, you do not worry when you are excited.

No time is better to start fulfilling your plans than now.

In past researches, the exercises that worked best as stress relievers for the general population are running, brisk walking, swimming and dancing. Heavy lifting is discouraged as it puts great stress on the body.

Journaling

One of the reasons why anxiety aggravates is because of the accumulation of worries and depression. When these harmful emotions are locked in, they fuel more negative emotions and become bigger over time as they pile up. According to studies, men have higher tendency to commit suicide and their lack of emotional connection with other people is one possible contributing factor.

Journaling is an adequate outlet for managing stress, disappointments and sadness. As you remove some emotional loads, you also feel lighter, which can help you think clearer. A journal also does not judge, so you can vent out everything you want to say without any worries of receiving prejudice.

All you have to do is write down your good and bad experiences for the day until you become comfortable in opening up even with an inanimate object. Psychotherapists believe that writing helps you train logical thinking as it is a natural process that your brain undergoes when doing this activity.

As your improvement becomes more significant as time goes by, start trying to open up with a real person as your next level. It will make you feel more comfortable and less paranoid with the people around you, which will also help you develop better self-esteem.

Laughter

Laughter yoga is gaining popularity because of the continuously increasing interest in the health benefits of laughter. To start off, people who laugh more often live longer by approximately 10 years. Their cells regenerate faster and their immune system is stronger. Overall wellness is important to keep you resistant to anxiety disorder and other mental problems, especially when you already manifest some physical symptoms at an early age.

When you laugh, the brain receives a signal to produce more endorphins and curb the secretion of cortisol, resulting in a positively effected mood (and more happiness). Since you receive a lot of positive mental pictures, you also have less time to entertain negative mental pictures that trigger anxiety attack. Can you imagine yourself actually suffering from an anxiety attack while watching a marathon of your favorite sitcom?

Hobby

A hobby is something that you really enjoy and occupy your time and mind. This is the perfect distraction for your uncontrollable worrying because you get to elicit good feelings, create happy thoughts and memories, and spend time on something worthwhile.

People with hobbies have lower stress-producing hormones called cortisol. This hormone is a major contributing factor in the development of anxiety disorders and depression, and the major cause of the symptoms of anxiety and panic attacks.

At the same time, they have higher secretion of endorphins, another hormone that is frequently called the "feel-good" hormone because of its effect on emotional and mental health. More endorphins in your body means having a happier life. It has also been associated with relaxation since trying to relax while having a boost of cortisol is basically impossible. No wonder it is hard to sleep and stay calm when you are having an anxiety attack and absorbing too much stress around you like while at work.

Sleep

Not just any sleep for that matter but a complete seven to eight hours of sleep every night. The length of sleep is important because the brain and body needs enough time to rest and regenerate. Unnecessary memories include pain, sadness, frustrations and minor details in your daily life that do not really have any meaning, such as the moment you flushed the toilet and opened the door, stay fresh in your mind unless you get sufficient rest.

Nature Tripping

Nature offers the basics of life, including peace, serenity and happiness. You can discover more about yourself while having a trip in nature than while conducting a self-evaluation in the isolated corner of your room. Nature does not give any distraction because everything you find there is a source of inspiration. Now even luxury spas incorporate nature elements to complete the relaxing atmosphere that they offer to their patrons.

Nature is a great antidote to anxiety and depression because most of their causes are man-made in nature, such as the trauma you had in a relationship or the car accident you were involved in. Stressors are also essentially man-made, which is a common result of modern living, fast-phase world, and insatiable demands.

Conclusion

Anxiety is a common problem which most of us are unaware of. I hope that with my book you were able to learn enough to address any anxiety issues you or your loved ones are having. Dealing with this disorder needs thorough understanding and enough support to achieve calm and relaxed mind. This books deals with the all the possible solutions to deal stress and to cope with daily challenges in life-the right to live a much more fulfilled life. By understanding what anxiety is, and how to properly treat it, you'll be one step closer to the life you've always dreamt of. No more having to deal with stress, or letting negative thoughts take over your decisions in life. I hope this book will give you the drive and motivation to be the person you've always wanted to be.

Life is tough and problems are always there to challenge us but this is not an excuse to succumb to it and lose all hope. It's written to inspire you to take life by the reins and actually make something out of yourself. If you feel like you've been held back in the past by your anxiety, it's time to empower yourself to take control over your life again. There will always be hope for those brave enough to take the next step.

I strive to make my future books better than the previous ones and one of the quickest ways to improve them is with feedback. Thank you in advance for your feedback.

About the Author

Nero Mayo is one of the multiple personalities of Bryan. Bryan is the Empire's Mastermind. The future Empire will create; Music and Movies, Kids T.V.-apps and much, much more. Nero Mayo publishes Ebooks on Kindle.

Author Central Page

http://www.amazon.com/Nero-Mayo-Michael/e/B01AZTQV4O/

Bryan, fresh out of the womb at 30-years-old has half the travelling experience already than half the people twice his age. He has done so many adventures he lost count at 3, but a small example of his time away from home involved travelling five days across the United States of America on a Greyhound bus (which he equates to breaking into the Professional Wrestling business), working on a Cruise line in Hawaii(which he equates to being taken hostage by a Sorority) and heading down under and working at a Grape Farm in Australia(which he equates to working at an Almond Factory in Australia). Besides "chillin' the freak out" Bryan loves self-expression through various mediums.

Check out the Digital version of this Ebook to get it in multiple languages, get free content instantly, join the email list and get a heads up of future releases!!

Also, you can check out all the other books released by Nero Mayo and Techyeah Productions!

Free Thank you Offers

I want to thank you again for checking out my book. I look forward to providing you with more of information that you can benefit from. Like I said at the beginning I want to have people, like you, that I notify when I'm putting out other valuable content!

http://www.amazon.com/Nero-Mayo-Michael/e/B01AZTQV4O/

Check out the author central page to see how you can join the email list and get TONS of free content and advance notifications of discounts on future releases!!

www.ingramcontent.com/pod-product-compliance
Lightning Source LLC
Chambersburg PA
CBHW071308280526
45788CB00004B/1856